Acknowledgement

The satisfactions, which accomplish a successful completion of any task, are incomplete without the mentioning of the names of those people who makes it possible.

We would never have been able to finish our book without you because "Coming together is a beginning. Keeping together is progress. Working together is success" and any successful task is not an individual's effort but it is a joint venture of many people who put in their mind and soul for the completion of that work.

We are pleased to express our deep sense of gratitude towards our parents for their creative suggestions, unfailing advice, and constant encouragement to transform teaching in the form of a user friendly book for the students.

We shall remain thankful to Hon. Management, Principal, all teaching and non-teaching staff members of P.S.G.V.P.M's College of Pharmacy, Shahada, Smt. S. S. Patil College of Pharmacy, Chopda & L. M. College of Pharmacy, Ahmedabad for encouraging us to write this book.

We also thanks to our colleagues and especially to Dr. V. R. Patil, BOS Chairmen of Pharmacognosy & Dr. R. Y. Chaudhari, BOS Member of Medicinal Chemistry, Kavayitri Bahinabai Chaudhari North Maharashtra University, Jalgaon, Maharashtra and Dr. P.R. Patil for helpful comments & suggestions.

We are thankful to Mr. Jignesh Furia Sir, Mr. Malik Shaikh, Mrs. Roshan Khan Madam, Chaitali Takle, Ravi Walodare and extend our thanks to supportive friends, colleagues for bringing out nicely printed book.

We hope this book will leave the desired impression and look forward to receive the comments from the readers.

Authors

A Practical Book of

MEDICINAL CHEMISTRY - III

As Per PCI Regulations

THIRD YEAR B. PHARM.
Semester VI

Dr. Sunila T. Patil
M. Pharm., Ph.D.
Associate Professor,
P.S.G.V.P.M's College of Pharmacy,
Shahada,
.

Dr. Md. Rageeb Md. Usman
M. Pharm., Ph.D., FAPP, FICPHS, FSRHCP, FRSH, FSPER
Associate Professor
Smt. S. S. Patil College of Pharmacy,
Chopda, Maharashtra,
Joint Secretaries, SPER Central Branch
and President, IPA/APP/RSH/SRHCP
Maharashtra State Branch

Dr. Parloop A. Bhatt
M. Pharm, Ph.D., DBM
Associate Professor
L. M. College of Pharmacy, Ahmedabad

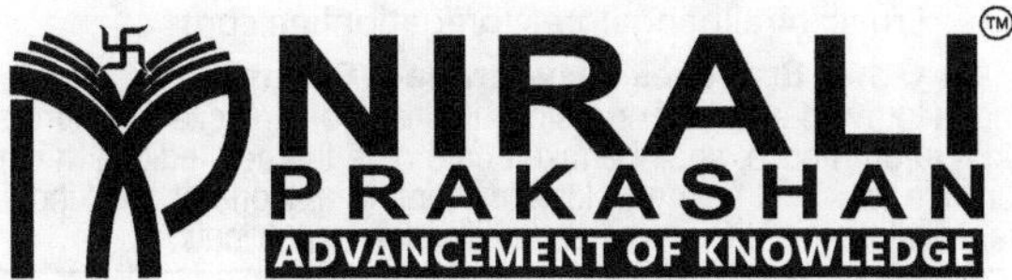

N4092

Medicinal Chemistry – III (Practical)   **ISBN 978-93-89686-75-3**

First Edition   :   **January 2020**

©   :   **Authors**

Published By :

NIRALI PRAKASHAN

Abhyudaya Pragati, 1312, Shivaji Nagar,

Off J.M. Road, PUNE – 411005

Tel - (020) 25512336/37/39, Fax - (020) 25511379

Email : niralipune@pragationline.com

➢ **DISTRIBUTION CENTRES**

PUNE

Nirali Prakashan   :   119, Budhwar Peth, Jogeshwari Mandir Lane, Pune 411002, Maharashtra
(For orders within Pune)   Tel : (020) 2445 2044, Mobile : 9657703145
Email : niralilocal@pragationline.com

Nirali Prakashan   :   S. No. 28/27, Dhayari, Near Asian College Pune 411041
(For orders outside Pune)   Tel : (020) 24690204 Fax : (020) 24690316; Mobile : 9657703143
Email : bookorder@pragationline.com

MUMBAI

Nirali Prakashan   :   385, S.V.P. Road, Rasdhara Co-op. Hsg. Society Ltd.,
Girgaum, Mumbai 400004, Maharashtra; Mobile : 9320129587
Tel : (022) 2385 6339 / 2386 9976, Fax : (022) 2386 9976
Email : niralimumbai@pragationline.com

➢ **DISTRIBUTION BRANCHES**

JALGAON

Nirali Prakashan   :   34, V. V. Golani Market, Navi Peth, Jalgaon 425001, Maharashtra,
Tel : (0257) 222 0395, Mob : 94234 91860; Email : niralijalgaon@pragationline.com

KOLHAPUR

Nirali Prakashan   :   New Mahadvar Road, Kedar Plaza, 1st Floor Opp. IDBI Bank, Kolhapur 416 012
Maharashtra. Mob : 9850046155; Email : niralikolhapur@pragationline.com

NAGPUR

Nirali Prakashan   :   Above Maratha Mandir, Shop No. 3, First Floor,
Rani Jhanshi Square, Sitabuldi, Nagpur 440012, Maharashtra
Tel : (0712) 254 7129; Email : niralinagpur@pragationline.com

DELHI

Nirali Prakashan   :   4593/15, Basement, Agarwal Lane, Ansari Road, Daryaganj
Near Times of India Building, New Delhi 110002 Mob : 08505972553
Email : niralidelhi@pragationline.com

BENGALURU

Nirali Prakashan   :   Maitri Ground Floor, Jaya Apartments, No. 99, 6th Cross, 6th Main,
Malleswaram, Bengaluru 560003, Karnataka; Mob : 9449043034
Email: niralibangalore@pragationline.com

Other Branches : Hyderabad, Chennai

niralipune@pragationline.com | www.pragationline.com

Also find us on 🅕 www.facebook.com/niralibooks

Preface

The subject emphasizes on the chemistry, mechanism of action, metabolism, adverse effects, Structure Activity Relationships (SAR), therapeutic uses and synthesis of important drugs.

Objectives: Upon completion of the course student should be able to:

1. Understand the importance of drug design and different techniques of drug design.

2. Understand the chemistry of drugs with respect to their biological activity.

3. Know the metabolism, adverse effects and therapeutic value of drugs.

4. Know the importance of SAR of drugs.

The efforts taken by authors to simplify the contents in a concise form to cater specially the needs of graduate students of pharmacy. The content of the book is restricted to the core and relevant part of the topic. For comprehensive learning, readers are expected to refer the reference books.

It is suggested that the students should develop habit of daily reading, writing structures so that confidence in the subject is built over a period of time.

We will be obliged to all teachers and students who will be kind enough to point out our mistakes that have escaped our attention.

Constructive suggestions, comments and criticism on the subject matter of the book will be gratefully acknowledged, as they will certainly help to improve future editions of the book. It is hoped that the book will be received favorably as an effective book by both students and teachers of pharmacy.

This book contains Question with answer after each Experiment for Exercise.

Authors

Syllabus

BP607P. MEDICINAL CHEMISTRY- III (Practical)

I. Preparation of Drugs and Intermediates

1. Sulphanilamide

2. 7-Hydroxy, 4-methyl coumarin

3. Chlorobutanol

4. Triphenyl imidazole

5. Tolbutamide

6. Hexamine

II. Assay of Drugs

1. Isonicotinic acid hydrazide

2. Chloroquine

3. Metronidazole

4. Dapsone

5. Chlorpheniramine maleate

6. Benzyl penicillin

III. Preparation of medicinally important compounds or intermediates by Microwave irradiation technique.

IV. Drawing structures and reactions using chemdraw®.

V. Determination of physicochemical properties such as log P, clog P, MR, Molecular weight, Hydrogen bond donors and acceptors for class of drugs course content using drug design software Drug likeliness screening (Lipinskies RO5).

****

SCHEMES FOR INTERNAL AND END EXAMINATIONS

Course Code	Name of the Course	Internal Assessment				End Semester Exams		Total Marks
		Continuous Mode	Sessional Exams		Total	Marks	Duration	
			Marks	Duration				
BP607P	Medicinal Chemistry-III (Practical)	05	10	4 Hrs.	15	35	4 Hrs	50

SCHEMES FOR CONTINUOUS MODE

Title	Marks
Attendance	2
Based on Practical Records, Regular viva voce, etc.	3
Total	**5**

GUIDELINES FOR ATTENDANCE MARKS

Percentage of Attendance	Practical
95 – 100	2
90 – 94	1.5
85 – 89	1
80 – 84	0.5
Less than 80	0

QUESTION PAPER PATTERN FOR SESSIONAL EXAMINATIONS

Title	Marks
Synopsis	10
Experiments	25
Viva voce	05
Total	40

Note: Sessional exam shall be conducted for 40 marks and shall be computed for 10 marks.

Title	Marks
Synopsis	05
Experiments	25
Viva voce	05
Total	35

GRADE POINT EQUIVALENT TO % OF MARK & PERFORMANCES

Percentage of Marks Obtained	Letter Grade	Grade Point	Performance
90.00 – 100	O	10	Outstanding
80.00 – 89.99	A	9	Excellent
70.00 – 79.99	B	8	Good
60.00 – 69.99	C	7	Fair
50.00 – 59.99	D	6	Average
Less than 50	F	0	Fail
Absent	AB	0	Fail

DECLARATION OF CLASS

Class	CGPA
First Class with Distinction	7.50 and above
First Class	6.00 to 7.49
Second Class	5.00 to 5.99

***

Contents

****

(I) PREPARATION OF DRUGS AND INTERMEDIATES

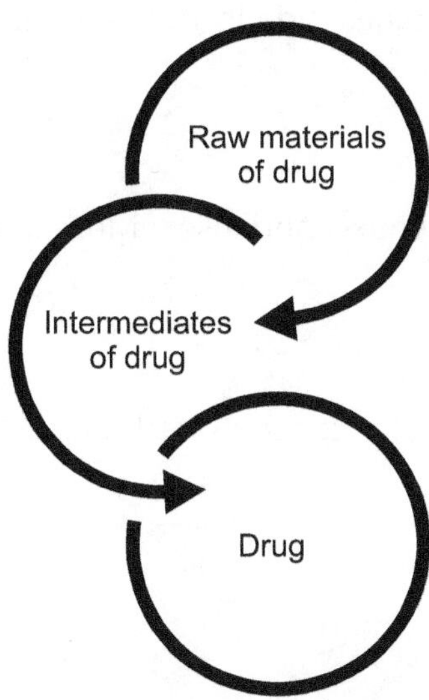

Chemical synthesis is the artificial execution of useful chemical reactions to obtain one or several products. This occurs by physical and chemical manipulations usually involving one or more reactions. In modern laboratory uses, the process is reproducible, reliable, and established to work the same in multiple laboratories.

A chemical synthesis involves one or more compounds known as reagents or reactants which will undergo a transformation when subjected to certain conditions. Various reaction types can be applied to formulate a desired product. This requires mixing the compounds in a reaction vessel, such as a chemical reactor or a simple round-bottom flask. Many reactions require some form of work-up or purification procedure to isolate the final product.

The amount of product produced in a chemical synthesis is the practical yield, which is typically expressed as a percentage conversion of the limiting reactant. Typically, practical yields are expressed as a weight in grams or as a percentage of the total theoretical quantity of product that could be produced based on the limiting reagent. A side reaction is an unwanted chemical reaction taking place, reducing the yield of the desired product.

***

Experiment No. 1

Aim: To prepare and submit Sulphanilamide from Acetanilide.

Requirements:

Apparatus:

Round bottom flask (RBF), Reflux condenser, Measuring cylinder, Beaker, Water bath, Buchner funnel.

Chemicals:

Acetanilide, Chlorosulphonic acid, concentrated ammonia, Dilute sulphuric acid, Sodium bicarbonate, concentrated hydrochloric acid.

Reactions:

Step 1:

Acetanilide + Chlorosulphonic acid $\longrightarrow$ p-acetamidobenzene sulphonyl chloride (SO_2Cl)

Step 2:

p-acetamidobenzene sulphonyl chloride (SO_2Cl) + NH_3 $\longrightarrow$ p-acetamidobenzene sulphonamide (SO_2NH_2)

Step 3:

p-acetamidobenzene sulphonamide (SO_2Cl) $\xrightarrow{H_3O^+}$ p-aminobenzene sulphonamide (Sulphanilamide) (SO_2NH_2)

Principle:

Sulphanilamide can be synthesized by taking acetanilide and react it with excess of chlorosulphonic acid, result in formation of p-acetamidobenzene sulphonyl chloride which readily converted into corresponding p-acetamidobenzene sulphonamides upon reaction with ammonia or ammonium carbonate. The acetamido groups undergo acid catalyzed hydrolysis reaction to form p-aminobenzene sulphonamide.

Procedure:

Step 1: Synthesis of p-acetamidobenzene sulphonyl chloride:

- Attach a double necked flask with a dropping funnel and a reflux condenser.
- Take 20 g of acetanilide in the flask and a chlorosulphonic acid, 50 ml (90 g) in the dropping funnel.
- Add the chlorosulphonic acid in small portions and shake the flask time to time to ensure thorough mixing. Heat the reaction mixture on a water bath for 1 hr.
- Keep it for some time for cooling and then pour the oily mixture into 300 g of crushed ice with stirring, contained in a 1 litre beaker.
- Carry out this operation in the fume cupboard since the excess of chlorosulphonic acid reacts vigorously with the water.
- Break up the lumps of solid material and mix the content by stirring for several min. in order to obtain an even suspension of the granular white solid.
- Filter off the p-acetamidobenzene sulphonyl chloride at the pump and wash it with a little cold water.
- Use the crude product in the next stage.

Step 2: Synthesis of p-acetamidobenzene sulphonamide:

- Transfer the crude p-acetamidobenzene sulphonyl chloride to the reaction flask and add a mixture of 70 ml of concentrated ammonia solution and 70 ml of water.
- Mix well the contents of the flask and heat the reaction mixture to just below the boiling point for about 15 minutes.
- The sulphonyl chloride will be converted into a pasty suspension of the corresponding sulphonamide.
- Cool the suspension product in ice, and then add dilute sulphuric acid until the mixture is just acidic to congo red paper.
- Collect the product on a Buchner funnel and wash with a little cold water.
- Dry the crude p-acetamidobenzene-sulphonamide at 100°C, the yield is about 18 g.

Step 3: Synthesis of p-aminobenzene sulphonamide:

- Transfer the crude p-acetamidobenzene sulphonamide to a 500 ml flask; mix 10 ml of concentrated hydrochloric acid 30 ml of water.
- Boil the mixture under reflux for 30-45 minutes.
- Then cool the solution to room temperature, if a solid separates, heat for a further some time.

- Treat the cooled solution with 2 g of charcoal, heat the mixture to boil and filter with suction.

- Place the filtrate of the mixture i.e. a solution of sulphanilamide hydrochloride in a one litre beaker and carefully add 16 g of solid sodium bicarbonate in some portions with constant stirring.

- After the evolution of gas, the suspension is test with litmus paper and if it is still acid, add more sodium bicarbonate until neutral. Cool in ice, filter off the sulphanilamide with suction.

- The yield is 15 g, m.p. 161-163°C. A pure product, m.p. 163-164°C, recrystallisation from water or from alcohol.

Calculation:

Here limiting reagent is acetanilide; hence yield should be calculated from its amount taken.

Molecular formula of acetanilide = C_8H_9NO

Molecular formula of sulphanilamide = $C_6H_8N_2O_2S$

Molecular weight of acetanilide = 135 g/mole

Molecular weight of sulphanilamide = 172 g/mole

Theoretical yield:

135 g acetanilide forms 172 g sulphanilamide

Therefore, 20 g acetanilide will form ....? (X) g sulphanilamide

X = (172 × 20)/135 = 25.48 g

Theoretical yield = 25.48 g

Practical yield = ————— g

% Yield = (Practical Yield/Theoretical Yield) × 100

Result:

Sulphanilamide was synthesized from acetanilide and submitted.

Name of compound	Sulphanilamide
Theoretical yield	...... gm
Practical yield	......gm
% Practical yield	...... %
Melting point	...... °C

VIVA-VOCE

1. Which acid is used in synthesis of Sulphanilamide?

Ans. Chlorosulfonic acid is used in synthesis of Sulphanilamide.

2. What are the uses of Sulphanilamide?

Ans. Sulfanilamide is used to treat vaginal yeast infections. Sulfanilamide reduces vaginal burning and itching. It works by stopping the growth of yeast that causes the infection.

3. What is the principle of synthesis of Sulphanilamide?

Ans. Sulphanilamide can be synthesized by taking acetanilide and react it with excess of chlorosulphonic acid, result in formation of p-acetamidobenzene sulphonyl chloride which readily converted into corresponding p-acetamidobenzene sulphonamides upon reaction with ammonia or ammonium carbonate. The acetamido groups undergo acid catalyzed hydrolysis reaction to form p-aminobenzene sulphonamide.

MULTIPLE CHOICE QUESTIONS

1. What is the molecular formula of Sulphanilamide?
   - (a) $C_6H_8N_2O_2S$
   - (b) $C_6H_{10}N_2O_2S$
   - (c) $C_6H_8NO_2S$
   - (d) $C_6H_{12}N_2O_2S$

2. What is the m.p of Sulphanilamide?
   - (a) 180-182°C
   - (b) 165-167 °C
   - (c) 195-197°C
   - (d) 244-246°C

3. Sulphanilamide is ....
   - (a) p-aminobenzene sulphonamide
   - (b) p-acetamidobenzene sulphonamide
   - (c) p-acetamidobenzene sulphonyl chloride
   - (d) p-acetamidosulphonamide

KEYS

1. (a)	2. (b)	3. (a)

****

Experiment No. 2

Aim: To prepare and submit 7-hydroxy-4-methyl coumarin from Resorcinol.

Requirements:

Apparatus:

Three necked flask, Thermometer, Mechanical stirrer, A dropping funnel, Beaker, Buchner funnel, Measuring cylinder.

Chemicals:

Concentrated sulphuric acid, Resorcinol, Ethyl acetoacetate, Sodium hydroxide solution (5%), Sulphuric acid (2 M), Ethanol (95%).

Reactions:

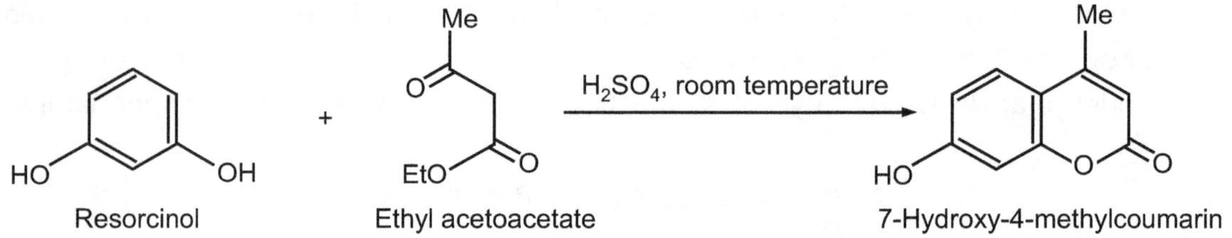

Resorcinol + Ethyl acetoacetate $\xrightarrow{\text{H}_2\text{SO}_4,\ \text{room temperature}}$ 7-Hydroxy-4-methylcoumarin

Mechanism:

The mechanism involves an esterification or transesterification followed by attack of the activated carbonyl ortho to the oxygen to generate the new ring. The final step is a dehydration, as seen in following aldol condensation.

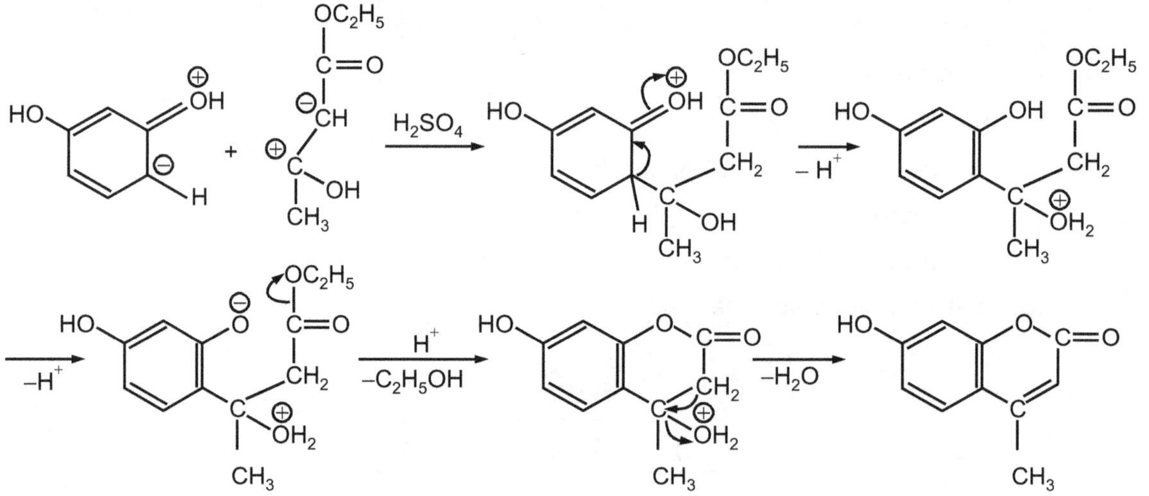

Principle:

A synthesis of coumarins involves the interaction of a phenol with a β-ketoester in presence of an acid condensing agent (Pechmann reaction). Concentrated sulphuric acid is used as the condensing agent for simple monohydric phenols and β-ketoesters, phenol itself reacts better in the presence of aluminium chloride. The mechanism of the reaction involve the initial formation of a β-hydroxy ester, which then cyclises and dehydrates to yield the coumarin.

Procedure:

- Take 1 litre of concentrated sulphuric acid in a 3 litres capacity 3 necked flask fitted with a thermometer, mechanical stirrer and a dropping funnel.

- Keep the flask in an ice bath.

- When the temperature falls below 10°C, add a solution of 100 g of resorcinol in 134 g (130.5 ml) of ethyl acetoacetate drop wise with stirring.

- Maintain the temperature below 10°C for 2 hours. Keep the mixture at room temperature for 18 hours and then pour it into crushed ice with vigorous stirring and 3 litres of water.

- Collect the precipitate by suction filtration and wash it with cold water.

- Dissolve the solid in 1500 ml of 5% sodium hydroxide solution, filter and add dilute 2 M sulphuric acid (about 550 ml) with vigorous stirring until the solution is acid to litmus.

- Filter the crude 4-methyl-7-hydroxycoumarin at the pump, wash with cold water and dry at 100°C.

- The yield is 155 g. Recrystallise from 95% ethanol: the pure compound separates in colourless crystals, m.p. 185°C.

Calculation:

Here limiting reagent is resorcinol; hence yield should be calculated from its amount taken.

Molecular formula of resorcinol = $C_6H_6O_2$

Molecular formula of 7-hydroxy-4-methyl coumarin = $C_{10}H_8O_3$

Molecular weight of resorcinol = 110 g/mole

Molecular weight of 7-hydroxy-4-methyl coumarin = 176 g/mole

Theoretical Yield:

110 g resorcinol forms 176 g 7-hydroxy-4-methyl coumarin

Therefore, 100 g resorcinol will form ....? (X) g 7-hydroxy-4-methyl coumarin

X = (176 × 100)/110 = g

Practical yield = ... g

% Yield = (Practical Yield/Theoretical Yield) × 100

Result:

7-hydroxy-4-methyl coumarin was synthesized from Resorcinol and submitted.

Name of compound	7-hydroxy-4-methyl coumarin
Theoretical yield	...... gm
Practical yield	...... gm
% Practical yield	...... %
Melting point	...... °C

VIVA-VOCE

1. Which phenol is used in synthesis of 7-hydroxy-4-methyl coumarin?

Ans. Resorcinol is used in synthesis of 7-hydroxy-4-methyl coumarin.

2. What are the uses of 7-hydroxy-4-methyl coumarin?

Ans. It is commercially used as laser dye. It is also used as the starting material for insecticide 'hymecromone.'

3. Which β-hydroxy ester is used in synthesis of 7-hydroxy-4-methyl coumarin?

Ans. Ethyl acetoacetate is used in synthesis of 7-hydroxy-4-methyl coumarin.

MULTIPLE CHOICE QUESTIONS

1. What is the molecular formula of 7-hydroxy-4-methyl coumarin?

   (a) $C_{10}H_8O_3$ (b) $C_8H_8O_3$

   (c) $C_{12}H_8NO_2S$ (d) $C_6H_{12}N_2O_2S$

2. What is the m.p of 7-hydroxy-4-methyl coumarin?

   (a) 185-187°C   (b) 165-167°C

   (c) 195-197°C   (d) 244-246°C

3. Synthesis of coumarins involves ...... condensation.

   (a) Pechmann   (b) Aldol

   (c) Claisen   (d) Phillips

KEYS

1. (a)	2. (a)	3. (a)

****

Experiment No. 3

Aim: To prepare and submit Chlorobutanol from Acetone.

Requirements:

Apparatus:

Beaker, Measuring cylinder, Mechanical stirrer, Ice bath, Buchner funnel.

Chemicals:

Acetone, Chloroform, Potassium hydroxide, Ethyl alcohol.

Reactions:

$$\underset{\text{Acetone}}{CH_3-CO-CH_3} + \underset{\text{Chloroform}}{CHCl_3} \xrightarrow{KOH} \underset{\text{Chlorobutanol}}{Cl_3C-C(OH)(CH_3)-CH_3}$$

Principle:

Chlorobutanol is synthesized by the addition of chloroform to acetone under the catalytic influence of powdered potassium hydroxide.

Procedure:

- The mixture of 50 g of acetone and 100 g of chloroform is cooled to below 0°C with continuously stirred.
- Add gradually 32.5 g of potassium hydroxide over a period of 6 hours. After it stand at room temperature for a further 3.6 hours with continuous stirring.
- The mass is filtered and the residue washed with acetone. The combined filtrates are distilled to recovered chloroform and acetone, and the fraction passing over between 165°C and 172°C is collected separately.
- The distillate is poured in water, and when this is complete the solid is filtered off and recrystallized from a mixture of alcohol and water.
- Chlorobutanol is extremely volatile even at ordinary temperatures.
- Chlorobutanol forms white glistening crystals. Chlorobutanol melts, when anhydrous, 96-97°C. Soluble in water and in 90% ethyl alcohol.

Calculation:

Here limiting reagent is acetone; hence yield should be calculated from it's amount taken.

Molecular formula of acetone = C_2H_6O

Molecular formula of chlorobutanol = $C_4H_7Cl_3O$

Molecular weight of acetone = 46 g/mole

Molecular weight of chlorobutanol = 177 g/mole

Theoretical yield:

46 g acetone forms 177 g chlorobutanol

Therefore, 50 g acetone will form ...... ? (X) g chlorobutanol

X = (177 × 50)/46 = g

Theoretical yield = g

Practical yield = ... g

% Yield = (Practical Yield/Theoretical Yield) × 100

Result:

Chlorobutanol was synthesized from acetone and submitted.

Name of compound	Chlorobutanol
Theoretical yield	...... gm
Practical yield	...... gm
% Practical yield	...... %
Melting point	...... °C

VIVA-VOCE

1. How Chlorobutanol is formed?

Ans. Chlorobutanol is formed by the reaction of chloroform and acetone in the presence of potassium or sodium hydroxide.

2. What are the uses of Chlorobutanol?

Ans. Chlorobutanol is used as a preservative, sedative, hypnotic and weak local anesthetic. It has antibacterial and antifungal properties.

MULTIPLE CHOICE QUESTIONS

1. What is the molecular formula of Chlorobutanol ?
   (a) $C_4H_6Cl_3O$ (b) $C_4H_7Cl_2O$
   (c) $C_4H_7Cl_3O$ (d) $C_4H_8Cl_3O$

2. What is the m.p of Chlorobutanol ?
   (a) 95-97°C   (b) 65-67°C
   (c) 195-197°C   (d) 125-127°C

3. IUPAC name of Chlorobutanol is ......
   (a) 2,2,2-Trichloro-2-methylpropan-2-ol
   (b) 1,1,1-Trichloro-2-methylpropan-2-ol
   (c) 1,1,1-Trichloro-2-methylpropan-3-ol
   (d) 2,2,2-Trichloro-2-methylethan-2-ol

KEYS

1. (c)	2. (a)	3. (b)

***

Experiment No. 4

Aim: To prepare and submit 2, 4, 5-Triphenyl Imidazole from Benzil.

Requirements:

Apparatus:

Round Bottom flask, Beaker, Measuring cylinder, Water bath, Buchner funnel.

Chemicals:

Benzil, Ammonium acetate, Benzaldehyde, Ethanol.

Reactions:

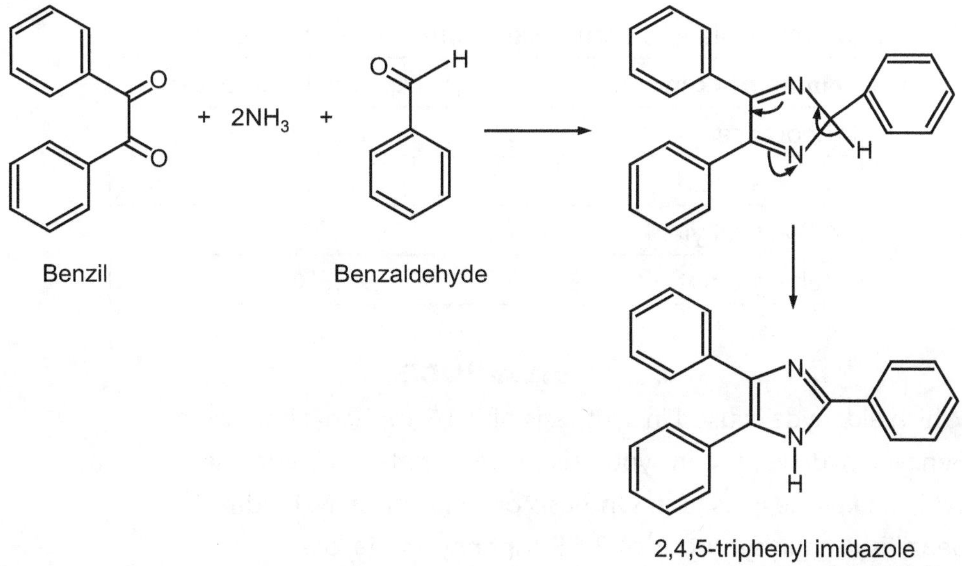

Benzil   + 2NH$_3$ +   Benzaldehyde   →

2,4,5-triphenyl imidazole

Principle:

Benzil reacts with benzaldehyde in presence of ammonium acetate results in formation of 2,4,5-triphenyl Imidazole.

Procedure:

- Take a solution of benzil (1.2 g), ammonium acetate (1.27 g) and benzaldehyde (20 ml) in glacial acetic acid and reflux for 2 hours.
- The reaction mixture to attain room temperature.
- Add 150 ml of water to that resulting solution and is filtered.
- The filtrate is neutralized with NH$_4$OH to give a solid pasty mass and filtered.
- Then solid mass is washed with toluene.
- Recrystallization is done with ethanol.

Calculation:

Here limiting reagent is Benzil; hence yield should be calculated from its amount taken.

Molecular formula of Benzil = C$_{14}$H$_{10}$O$_2$

Molecular formula of 2, 4, 5-triphenyl imidazole = C$_{21}$H$_{16}$N$_2$

Molecular weight of Benzil = 210 g/mole

Molecular weight of 2, 4, 5-triphenyl imidazole = 296 g/mole

Theoretical yield:

210 g Benzil forms 296 g 2, 4, 5-triphenyl imidazole

Therefore, 1.2 g Benzil will form ....? (X) g 2,4,5-triphenyl Imidazole

X = (296 × 1.2)/210 = 1.69 g

Theoretical yield = 1.69 g

Practical yield = ... g

% Yield = (Practical Yield/Theoretical Yield) × 100

Result:

2, 4, 5-triphenyl Imidazole was synthesized from Benzil and submitted.

Name of compound	2,4,5-triphenyl Imidazole
Theoretical yield	...... gm
Practical yield	...... gm
% Practical yield	...... %
Melting point	...... °C

VIVA-VOCE

1.　Which aldehyde is used in synthesis of 2,4,5-triphenyl imidazole?

Ans.　Benzaldehyde is used in synthesis of 2,4,5-triphenyl imidazole.

2.　Which diketone is used in synthesis of 2,4,5-triphenyl imidazole?

Ans.　Benzil is used in synthesis of 2,4,5-triphenyl imidazole.

3.　Give the principle of synthesis of 2,4,5-triphenyl imidazole?

Ans.　Benzil reacts with benzaldehyde in presence of ammonium acetate results in formation of 2,4,5-triphenyl Imidazole.

MULTIPLE CHOICE QUESTIONS

1.　What is the molecular formula of 2,4,5-triphenyl imidazole?

　(a)　$C_{21}H_{16}N_2$　　　　　　　　　(b)　$C_6H_{10}N_2O_2$

　(c)　$C_{16}H_{18}NO_2$　　　　　　　　　(d)　$C_{21}H_{18}N_2$

2.　What is the molecular weight of 2,4,5-triphenyl Imidazole?

　(a)　220 g/mol　　　　　　　　　(b)　296 g/mole

　(c)　242 g/mol　　　　　　　　　(d)　252 g/mol

KEYS

1. (a)	2. (b)

***

Experiment No. 5

Aim: To prepare and submit Tolbutamide from *p*-toluene sulfonamide.

Requirements:

Apparatus:

Round Bottom flask, Reflux condenser, Beaker, Measuring cylinder, Water bath, Buchner funnel.

Chemicals:

p-toluene sulfonamide, Butyl isocyanate, Acetone, Potassium carbonate.

Reactions:

p-toluene sulfonamide　　　Butyl isocyanate　　　　　　　　Tolbutamide

Principal:

Tolbutamide can be prepared by condensation of the toluene-p-sulfonamide with n-butyl isocyanate followed by acidification.

Procedure:

- p-toluene sulfonamide treated with butyl isocyanate in presence of acetone and potassium carbonate.
- Reflux it for 18 hours to produce tolbutamide.
- Recrystallize it to form dilute ethanol.

Calculation:

Here limiting reagent is p-toluene sulfonamide; hence yield should be calculated from its amount taken.

Molecular formula of *p*-toluene sulfonamide = $C_7H_9O_2NS$

Molecular formula of Tolbutamide = $C_{12}H_{18}O_3N_2S$

Molecular weight of *p*-toluene sulfonamide = 171 g/mole

Molecular weight of Tolbutamide = 270 g/mole

Theoretical yield:

171 g p-toluenesulfonamide forms 270 g Tolbutamide

Therefore, 1 g p-toluene sulfonamide will form ...... ? (X) g Tolbutamide

X = (270 × 1) / 171 = 1.58 g

Theoretical yield = g

Practical yield = 1.58 g

% Yield = (Practical Yield/Theoretical Yield) × 100

Result:

Tolbutamide was synthesized from p-toluene sulfonamide and submitted.

Name of compound	Tolbutamide
Theoretical yield	...... gm
Practical yield	...... gm
% Practical yield	...... %
Melting point	...... °C

VIVA-VOCE

1. What are the uses of Tolbutamide?

Ans. Tolbutamide is used to treat type 2 diabetes. It also helps the body use insulin efficiently.

2. What is the principal of Tolbutamide synthesis?

Ans. Tolbutamide can be made by condensation of the toluene-p-sulfonamide with n-butyl isocyanate followed by acidification.

MULTIPLE CHOICE QUESTIONS

1. What is the molecular formula of Tolbutamide?
   (a) $C_{12}H_{18}O_3N_2S$ 　　　　　　　(b) $C_{10}H_{18}O_3N_2S$
   (c) $C_{12}H_8NO_2S$ 　　　　　　　　(d) $C_6H_{12}N_2O_2S$

2. What is the m.p of Tolbutamide?
   (a) 155-157°C 　　　　　　　　　(b) 185-187°C
   (c) 128-130°C 　　　　　　　　　(d) 244-246°C

3. *Tolbutamide* is a first-generation ...... channels blocker?
   (a) Sodium 　　　　　　　　　　(b) Chloride
   (c) Potassium 　　　　　　　　　(d) Calcium

KEYS

1. (a)	2. (c)	3. (c)

***

Experiment No. 6

Aim: To prepare and submit Hexamine from Formaldehyde.

Requirements:

Apparatus:

Round Bottom flask, Beaker, Measuring cylinder, Water bath, Buchner funnel.

Chemicals:

Formaldehyde, Ammonium hydroxide, Ammonia, Ethyl alcohol.

Reactions:

$$6CH_2O + 6NH_3 \longrightarrow \text{Hexamine} + 6H_2O$$

Formaldehyde   Ammonia   Hexamine

Principle:

Hexamine is synthesized by the condensation of formaldehyde and ammonia.

Procedure:

- 47.3 g of a 38% formaldehyde solution is reacted with 70 g of 20% ammonium hydroxide solution, until the solution is slightly alkaline.
- The mixture is allowed to stand at room temperature for several hours and if necessary more ammonia being added.
- The solution is filtered and then evaporated to a thick paste.
- The hexamine crystals are filtered and washed with ethyl alcohol.
- The pure hexamine is recrystallized from water or alcohol.

Calculation:

Here limiting reagent is formaldehyde; hence yield should be calculated from its amount taken.

Molecular formula of formaldehyde = CH_2O

Molecular formula of hexamine = $C_6H_6N_4$

Molecular weight of formaldehyde = 30 g/mole

Molecular weight of hexamine = 134 g/mole

Theoretical yield:

30 g formaldehyde forms 134 g hexamine

Therefore, 47.3 g formaldehyde will form ...... ? (X) g hexamine

X = (134 × 47.3)/30 = g

Theoretical yield = g

Practical yield = ... g

% Yield = (Practical Yield/Theoretical Yield) × 100

Result:

Hexamine was synthesized from formaldehyde and submitted.

Name of compound	Hexamine
Theoretical yield	...... gm
Practical yield	...... gm
% Practical yield	...... %
Melting point	...... °C

VIVA-VOCE

1.　Which aldehyde is used in synthesis of Hexamine?

Ans.　Formaldehyde is used in synthesis of Hexamine.

2.　What are the uses of Hexamine?

Ans.　Hexamine is used for the treatment, control, prevention and improvement of the Gastro-urinary infections and Urinary tract infections.

3.　What is the principle of synthesis of Hexamine?

Ans.　Hexamine is synthesized by the condensation of formaldehyde and ammonia.

MULTIPLE CHOICE QUESTIONS

1.　What is the molecular formula of Hexamine?

(a)　$C_6H_6N_4$　　　　　　　　(b)　$C_6H_6N_3$

(c)　$C_6H_6N_2$　　　　　　　　(d)　C_6H_6N

2.　What is the melting point of Hexamine?

(a)　180-182°C　　　　　　　　(b)　280-282°C

(c)　195-197°C　　　　　　　　(d)　244-246°C

3.　Hexamine is ......

(a)　Hexamethylenetetramine　　　　(b)　Hexamethylenetriamine

(c)　Hexamethyleneamine　　　　　(d)　Hexamethylenediamine

KEYS

1. (a)	2. (b)	3. (a)

***

(II) ASSAY OF DRUGS

Assay is a procedure for the examination or determination of quality or strength of a substance. It is the analysis of the amount of metal in an ore, or the determination of the amount of purities in a precious metal. An assay procedure is generally employed to evaluate an intensive property of the measured entity, called "analyte". It is expressed in a relevant measurement unit like density, molarity, etc.

A chemical assay refers to the analysis of a sample material, called analyte, using a set of chemical procedures.

- Qualitative - extraction, distillation, precipitation and other methods that determine physicochemical properties.

- Quantitative - volume or weight of the substance.

Characteristics of Good Assay Method: Sensitivity, Specificity, Repeatability, Reproducibility, Validity.

✱✱✱

Experiment No. 7

Aim: To carry out the assay of Isonicotinic acid hydrazide (Isoniazid) Tablets IP.

Requirements:

Apparatus:

Volumetric flask, Measuring cylinder, Analytical balance, Weight box, Beaker, Burette, Conical flask and UV Spectrometer.

Chemicals:

Isoniazid tablets, Potassium bromate, Methyl red, Dimethyl formamide, Sodium carbonate, Sodium thiosulfate, Starch solution.

Principle:

The reaction is between isoniazid and potassium bromine, but solution of bromine is not stable. Therefore, a small amount of potassium bromide is added to the acidified solution of isoniazid, which is slowly titrated with potassium bromated. The reaction between $KBrO_3$, KBr, HCl, liberate bromine and this bromine oxidizes isoniazid. At the end point when HCl get deflected, changes colour from red to yellow.

Preparation and Standardization of standard solutions:

1. Preparation of Potassium Bromate, 0.0167 M:

Dissolve 2.783 gm of potassium bromate in sufficient water to produce 1000 ml.

2. Preparation of Sodium Thiosulphate, xM:

Dissolve 248x g of Sodium thiosulphate and 2x g of sodium carbonate in sufficient water to produce 1000 ml.

3. Standardization of Potassium Bromate:

Transfer the volume of about 30 ml of potassium bromate into a glass stoppered flask, add 3 ml of potassium iodide, following by 3 ml of hydrochloric acid. Allow to stand for five minutes at room temperature, then titrate the liberated iodine with standard sodium thiosulphate by using 3 ml of starch solution as an indicator. Collect for a blank on the same quantities of the same reagents. Each ml of 0.1 N sodium thiosulphate is equivalent to 0.002784 gm of potassium bromate.

Procedure:

1. Assay Method by Volumetric Analysis:

- Weigh and powder 20 tablets.
- Weigh accurately quantity of the powder equivalent to 0.4 g of isoniazid and dissolve in water, filter and wash the residue with sufficient water to produce 250 ml.
- Add 50 ml of water to 50 ml of the resulting solution, 20 ml of hydrochloric acid and 0.2 g of potassium bromide.
- Titrate slowly with 0.0167 M potassium bromate with continuous shaking using 0.05 ml of methyl red solution as indicator, until the red colour disappears.
- Each ml of 0.0167 M potassium bromate is equivalent to 0.003429 g of $C_6H_7N_3O$.

2. Assay Method by UV-Spectroscopic Method:

- Weigh about 80 mg of isoniazid and add 150 ml of dimethyl formamide, then add sufficient water to produce 500 ml.
- Dilute 5 ml to 100 ml with water and mix. Measure the absorbance of the resulting solution at the maximum at about 367 nm.
- Calculate the content of $C_8H_7N_3O_5$ taking 750 as the specific absorbance at 367 nm.

Result:

The given sample contains …… mg of isoniazid.

VIVA-VOCE

1. How will you prepare Sodium Thiosulphate, 0.1 N?

Ans. Solution of any normality 0.1 N is prepared by dissolving 24.8 g of sodium thiosulphate and 0.2 g of sodium carbonate in sufficient carbon dioxide free water to produce 1000 ml.

2. What are the uses of Isoniazid?

Ans. Isoniazid is used in tuberculosis (TB) infections.

3. Write down the factor involve in assay of Isoniazid?

Ans. Each ml of 0.0167 M potassium bromate is equivalent to 0.003429 g of $C_6H_7N_3O$.

MULTIPLE CHOICE QUESTIONS

1. Which indicator is used in assay of Isoniazid?
   - (a) Phenol red
   - (b) Methyl red
   - (c) Phenolphthalein
   - (d) Methyl orange
2. Molecular weight of Isoniazid is ……
   - (a) 137.142 g
   - (b) 119.55 g
   - (c) 318.86 g
   - (d) 388.85 g

KEYS

1. (b)	2. (d)

***

Experiment No. 8

Aim: To carry out the assay of Chloroquine IP.

Requirements:

Apparatus:

Volumetric flask, Measuring cylinder, Analytical balance, Weight box, Beaker, Burette and Conical flask.

Chemicals:

Perchloric acid, Anhydrous glacial acetic acid.

Principle:

It involves non-aqueous potentiometric titration with perchloric acid as titrant.

Preparation of Perchloric acid, 0.1 M:

Mix 8.5 ml of perchloric acid with 500 ml of anhydrous glacial acetic acid and 25 ml of acetic anhydride, cool and add anhydrous glacial acetic acid to produce 1000 ml. The prepared solution is allowed to stand for 1 day and again titrate the water content. The solution so obtained should contain between 0.02% and 0.05% of water.

Standardization of 0.1 M Perchloric acid:

Weigh accurately about 0.35 gm of Potassium hydrogen phthalate and dissolve in 50 ml of anhydrous glacial acetic acid. Add 0.1 ml of crystal violet solution as on indicator and titrate with the perchloric acid solution until the violet colour changes to emerald-green. Perform a blank determination. Each ml of 0.1 M perchloric acid is equivalent to 0.02042 g of $C_8H_5KO_4$.

Procedure:

- Weigh accurately about 0.5 gm of Chloroquine.
- Dissolve it in 50 ml of anhydrous glacial acetic acid and carry out Method A for non-aqueous titration, determining the end-point potentiometrically.
- Perform a blank determination.
- Each ml of 0.1 M Perchloric acid is equivalent to 0.0418 g of $C_{18}H_{26}ClN_3, H_2SO_4$.

Non-Aqueous Titration:

Method A:

Dissolve the prescribed quantity of the substance in a suitable volume of anhydrous glacial acetic acid, prepare a solution as directed in the monograph and determine the equivalence point potentiometrically using 0.1 M Perchloric acid as titrant. Potentiometric titration may be carried out using a glass electrode and a standard reference electrode, e.g. Calomel reference electrode containing saturated solution of potassium chloride in water. Potentiometric titrations may also be carried out by using a glass electrode and a saturated solution of potassium chloride in water has been replaced by a saturated solution of potassium chloride in methanol. Alternatively, a combined electrode may be used.

Result:

The given sample contains ...... mg of Chloroquine.

VIVA-VOCE

1.   Which titrant is used in assay of Chloroquine?

Ans. 0.1 M Perchloric acid is used as titrant in assay of Chloroquine.

2.   What are the uses of Chloroquine?

Ans. Chloroquine is used to prevent or treat malaria.

3.   Which indicator is used in standardization of 0.1 M Perchloric acid?

Ans. Crystal violet indicator is used in standardization of 0.1 M Perchloric acid.

MULTIPLE CHOICE QUESTIONS

1.   Assay of Chloroquine is a .... type of titration?

    (a)   Aqueous   (b)   Non-aqueous

    (c)   Complexometry   (d)   Iodometry

2.   What is the molecular formula of Chloroquine?

    (a) $C_{18}H_{26}ClN_3$ (b) $C_{16}H_{24}ClN_2$

    (c) $C_{14}H_{26}ClN_2$ (d) $C_{18}H_{24}ClN_3$

KEYS

1. (b)	2. (a)

***

Experiment No. 9

Aim: To carry out the assay of Metronidazole Tablets.

Requirements:

Apparatus:

Volumetric flask, Measuring cylinder, Analytical balance, Weight box, Beaker, Burette and Conical flask.

Chemicals:

Metronidazole tablets, 0.1 N Perchloric acid, Anhydrous glacial acetic acid, Brilliant green, Potassium hydrogen phthalate and Crystal violet.

Principle:

Metronidazole tablets are assayed by non-aqueous titration in which the tertiary amine group is titrated with perchloric acid using brilliant green as indicator.

Preparation of Perchloric acid, 0.1 M:

Mix 8.5 ml of perchloric acid with 500 ml of anhydrous glacial acetic acid and 25 ml of acetic anhydride, cool and add anhydrous glacial acetic acid to produce 1000 ml. The prepared solution is allowed to stand for 1 day and again titrate the water content. The solution so obtained should contain between 0.02% and 0.05% of water.

Weigh accurately about 0.35 gm of Potassium hydrogen phthalate and dissolve in 50 ml of anhydrous glacial acetic acid. Add 0.1 ml of crystal violet solution as indicator and titrate with the perchloric acid solution until the violet colour changes to emerald-green. Perform a blank determination. Each ml of 0.1 M Perchloric acid is equivalent to 0.02042 g of $C_8H_5KO_4$.

Procedure:

- Weigh and powder of 20 tablets of Metronidazole.
- Weigh accurately a quantity of the powder containing about 0.2 g of Metronidazole, transfer to a glass crucible and extract with six quantities, each of 10 ml, of hot acetone.
- Cool it and add 50 ml of acetic anhydride to the combined extracts.
- Titrate with 0.1 M Perchloric acid, using 0.1 ml of 1% w/v solution of brilliant green in anhydrous glacial acetic acid as indicator to a yellowish-green end point. Carry out a blank titration.
- Each ml of 0.1 M Perchloric acid is equivalent to 0.01712 g of $C_6H_9N_3O_3$.

Result:

The given sample contains …… mg of Metronidazole.

VIVA-VOCE

1. Which titrant is used in assay of Metronidazole?

Ans. 0.1 M Perchloric acid is used as titrant in assay of Metronidazole.

2. What are the uses of Metronidazole?

Ans. Atropine sulfate is an antimuscarinic agent used to treat bradycardia, reduce salivation and bronchial secretions before surgery, also used as an antidote for overdose of cholinergic drugs or mushroom poisoning.

MULTIPLE CHOICE QUESTIONS

1. Which indicator is used in assay of Metronidazole?

   (a) Phenol red　　　　　　　　　(b) Methyl red

   (c) Brilliant green　　　　　　　(d) Methyl orange

2. Assay of Metronidazole is a ...... type of titration?

   (a) Aqueous　　　　　　　　　　(b) Non-aqueous

   (c) Complexometry　　　　　　　(d) Iodometry

KEYS

1. (c)	2. (b)	3. ()

***

Experiment No. 10

Aim: To carry out the assay of Dapsone Tablet IP.

Requirements:

Apparatus:

Volumetric flask, Measuring cylinder, Analytical balance, Weight box, Beaker, Burette and Conical flask.

Chemicals:

Sodium nitrite, Hydrochloric acid and Dapsone tablets.

Principle:

Assay of dapsone involves diazotization titration. Primary aromatic amines react with sodium nitrite in acid solution to form diazonium salts. The end point in this titration method is located by using starch iodide paste as indicator. A small amount of iodide included in the titration mixture is converted to iodine by excess of nitrous acid, this is detected using starch indicator.

Procedure:

- Weigh and powder 20 tablets of Dapsone.
- Weigh accurately a quantity of the powder equivalent to 0.25 g of dapsone and dissolve in mixture of 15 ml of water and 15 ml of 2 M hydrochloric acid.
- Cool the solution to about 15°C.
- Carry out the nitrite titration.
- Perform a blank determination.
- Each ml of 0.1M sodium nitrite is equivalent to 0.01242 g of $C_{12}H_{12}N_2O_2S$.

Result:

The given sample contains …… mg of dapsone.

VIVA-VOCE

1. What are the uses of Dapsone?

Ans. Dapsone is an antibacterial in the sulfone family of *antibiotics*. It is used to treat leprosy and the skin condition known as dermatitis herpetiformis.

2. What is the principle of assay of Dapsone?

Ans. Assay of dapsone involves diazotization titration.

3. Write down the factor involve in assay of Dapsone?

Ans. Each ml of 0.1M sodium nitrite is equivalent to 0.01242 g of $C_{12}H_{12}N_2O_2S$.

MULTIPLE CHOICE QUESTIONS

1. Which indicator is used in assay of Dapsone?

    (a) Phenol red   (b) Bromothymol blue

    (c) Phenolphthalein   (d) Starch iodide paste

2. What is the molecular formula of Dapsone?

    (a) $C_{12}H_{12}N_2O_2S$ (b) $C_{10}H_{12}N_2O_2S$

    (c) $C_{12}H_{14}N_2O_2S$ (d) $C_{10}H_{10}N_2O_2S$

KEYS

1. (d)	2. (a)

***

Experiment No. 11

Aim: To carry out the assay of Chlorpheniramine Maleate IP.

Requirements:

Apparatus:

Volumetric flask, Measuring cylinder, Analytical balance, Weight box, Beaker, Burette and Conical flask.

Chemicals:

Perchloric acid, Anhydrous glacial acetic acid, Chlorpheniramine Maleate.

Principle:

It is a non-aqueous titration.

Preparation of Perchloric acid, 0.1 M:

Mix 8.5 ml of perchloric acid with 500 ml of anhydrous glacial acetic acid and 25 ml of acetic anhydride then cool it and add anhydrous glacial acetic acid to produce 1000 ml. Allow the prepared solution to stand for 1 day and titrate the water content.

Standardization of 0.1 M Perchloric acid:

Weigh accurately about 0.35 gm of Potassium hydrogen phthalate and dissolve it in 50 ml of anhydrous glacial acetic acid. Add 0.1 ml of crystal violet solution as indicator and titrate with the perchloric acid solution until the violet colour changes to emerald-green. Perform a blank determination. Each ml of 0.1 M Perchloric acid is equivalent to 0.02042 g of $C_8H_5KO_4$.

Procedure:

- Weigh accurately about 0.2 gm of Chlorpheniramine Maleate and dissolve in 20 ml of anhydrous glacial acetic acid.
- Carry out method A for non-aqueous titration.
- Determining the end point potentiometrically.
- Perform a blank determination.
- Each ml of 0.1 M perchloric acid is equivalent to 0.01954 g of $C_{16}H_{19}ClN_2, C_4H_4O_4$.

Non-Aqueous Titration:

Method A:

Dissolve the prescribed quantity of the substance in a suitable volume of anhydrous glacial acetic acid or prepare a solution as directed in the monograph and determine the equivalence point potentiometrically using 0.1 M Perchloric acid as titrant. Potentiometric titration may be carried out using a glass electrode and a standard reference electrode, e.g. Calomel reference electrode containing saturated solution of potassium chloride in water. Potentiometric titrations may also be carried out by using a glass electrode and a saturated solution of potassium chloride in water has been replaced by a saturated solution of potassium chloride in methanol. Alternatively, a combined electrode may be used. The junction between the Calomel electrode and the titration liquid should have a reasonably low electrical resistance. The connections between the potentiometer and the electrode system must be made according to the manufacturer's instructions to avoid problems of instability.

Result:

The given sample contains …… mg of Chlorpheniramine Maleate.

VIVA-VOCE

1. What is the principle of assay of Chlorpheniramine Maleate?

Ans. It is a non-aqueous titration.

2. What are the uses of Chlorpheniramine Maleate?

Ans. Chlorpheniramine maleate is used as an antihistaminic agents, which relieve symptoms of allergy, fever and the common cold.

3. Write down the factor involved in assay of Chlorpheniramine Maleate?

Ans. Each ml of 0.1 M perchloric acid is equivalent to 0.01954 g of $C_{16}H_{19}ClN_2, C_4H_4O_4$.

MULTIPLE CHOICE QUESTIONS

1. …… titrant is used in assay of Chlorpheniramine Maleate?
    (a) 0.1 M Nitric acid   (b) 0.1 M Hydrochloric acid
    (c) 0.1 M Perchloric acid   (d) 0.1 M Sodium hydroxide

2. Which indicator is used in standardization of 0.1 M Perchloric acid?
    (a) Phenol red   (b) Bromothymol blue
    (c) Phenolphthalein   (d) Crystal violet

KEYS

1. (c)	2. (d)

****

Experiment No. 12

Aim: To carry out the assay of Benzyl Penicillin Potassium IP.

Requirements:

Apparatus:

Volumetric flask, Measuring cylinder, Analytical balance, Weight box, Beaker, Pipette, Burette and Conical flask.

Chemicals:

1 M nitric acid, 1 M Sodium hydroxide, 0.02 M mercuric nitrate, Benzyl Penicillin Potassium.

Preparation and Standardization of Standard Solutions:

1. **Preparation of Sodium hydroxide, xM:** Solutions of any molarity xM may be prepared by dissolving 40x g of Sodium hydroxide in sufficient water to produce 1000 ml.

2. **Preparation of Nitric Acid, xM:** Solutions of any molarity xM may be prepared by diluting 63x ml of nitric acid to 1000 ml with water.

3. **Preparation of Acetate Buffer, pH 4.6:** Dissolve 5.4 gm of sodium acetate in 50 ml of water, then add 2.4 ml of glacial acetic acid. Diluted the resulting solution with water to 100 ml and adjust the pH if necessary.

4. **Preparation of Mercuric Nitrate, 0.02 M:** Dissolve 6.85 g of mercuric nitrate in 20 ml of 1 M nitric acid and add sufficient water to produce 1000 ml.

5. **Standardization of Mercuric Nitrate, 0.02 M:** Dissolve 15 mg of sodium chloride in 100 ml of water and titrate it with the mercuric nitrate solution. Determine the end point potentiometrically, using a platinum or mercury indicator electrode and a mercury-mercurous sulphate reference electrode.

    Each ml of 0.02 M mercuric nitrate is equivalent to 0.002338 g of NaCl.

Procedure:

*   Weigh accurately about 50 mg of Benzyl Penicillin Potassium, dissolve in 5 ml of water and add 5 ml of 1 M sodium hydroxide solution. Allow to stand for 15 minutes.

*   Add 5 ml of 1 M nitric acid, 20 ml of acetate buffer pH 4.5 and 20 ml of water and titrating at 35-40°C with 0.02 M mercuric nitrate.

*   Determine the end–point potentiometrically using a platinum or mercury indicator electrode and a mercury-mercurous sulphate reference electrode.

- Each ml of 0.002 M mercuric nitrate is equivalent to 0.007450 g of total penicillins, calculated as $C_{16}H_{17}KN_2O_4S$.
- To 0.25 g, accurately weighed, add 25 ml of water and 25 ml of acetate buffer pH 4.6 and shake until solution is complete. Titrate immediately at room temperature with 0.02 M mercuric nitrate determining the end-point as above.
- Each ml of 0.02 M mercuric nitrate is equivalent to 0.007450 g of degradation products, calculated as $C_{16}H_{17}KN_2O_4S$.
- Calculate the percentage content of total penicillins and the percentage content of degradation products.
- The difference between the two percentages is the content of penicillins.

Result:

The given sample contains ...... mg of Benzyl Penicillin.

VIVA-VOCE

1. How will you prepared 0.1 M NaOH?

Ans. 0.1 M NaOH is prepared by dissolving 4 g of Sodium hydroxide in sufficient water to produce 1000 ml.

2. What are the uses of Benzyl Penicillin?

Ans. Benzyl Penicillin is used as an antibiotic to treat a bacterial infections such as pneumonia, strep throat, syphilis, diphtheria, tetanus etc.

3. How will you prepared Mercuric Nitrate 0.02 M?

Ans. Dissolve 6.85 g of mercuric nitrate in 20 ml of 1 M nitric acid and add sufficient water to produce 1000 ml.

MULTIPLE CHOICE QUESTIONS

1. Which Buffer is used in assay of Benzyl Penicillin?
   - (a) Acetate buffer
   - (b) Citrate buffer
   - (c) Bicarbonate buffer
   - (d) Phosphate buffer

2. ...... is used for standardization of 0.02 M mercuric nitrate?
   - (a) NaCl
   - (b) KOH
   - (c) NaBr
   - (d) KBr

KEYS

1. (a)	2. (a)

***

(III) PREPARATION OF MEDICINALLY IMPORTANT COMPOUNDS OR INTERMEDIATES BY MICROWAVE IRRADIATION TECHNIQUE

Microwave organic synthesis opens up new opportunities to the synthetic chemist in the form of new reaction that are not possible by conventional heating and serve a flexible platform for chemical reaction. The time saved by using focused microwaves is potentially important in traditional organic synthesis but could be of even greater importance in high-speed combinatorial and medicinal chemistry. The study presents examples that demonstrate the significance of these advantages to industrial application.

The promotion of microwave assisted reactions in organic chemistry has improved the speed, reduced cost, reduced energy.

Advantages of Microwaves:

   (i)   Rapid reactions.

   (ii)   High purity of products.

   (iii) Less side-product.

   (iv)   Improved yields.

   (v)   Simplified and improved synthetic procedure.

   (vi)   Wider usable range of temperature.

   (vii) Higher energy efficiency.

  (viii) Sophisticated measurement and safety technology.

   (ix)   Modular systems enable changing from mg to kg scale.

Disadvantages of Microwaves:

   (i)   Heat force control is difficult.

   (ii)   Water evaporation.

   (iii) Closed container is dangerous because it could be burst.

Principles of Microwave Activation:

In the electromagnetic spectrum the microwave radiation region is located between infrared radiation andradio-waves.

✳✳✳

Experiment No. 13

Aim: Synthesis of Phenytoin (Benzillic acid rearrangement).

Benzil   Urea   5,5 - diphenyl hydantoin

A mixture 2.0 gm of benzil, 1.13 gm of urea and ethanol were taken in a 250 ml round botton flask. 30% NaOH solution was added to that flask and the reaction was subjected to microwave at 160 watts for 30 minutes. Reaction mixture was rendered acidic with concentrated HCl. The product obtained was separated by filtration at the pump and washed with alcohol. Melting point is 296-298°C.

****

Experiment No. 14

Aim: Synthesis of Tetrahydro pyrimidine (Bignelli Condensation).

Benzaldehyde   Ethylacetoacetate   Urea   Substituted pyrimidine

An equimolar mixture of aromatic aldehyde, ethylacetocaetate and urea were taken in a 250 ml round botton flask. To this few drops of concentrated hydrochloric acid is added as catalyst. The reaction was subjected to microwave at 180 watts and monitored on TLC for 30 seconds. After 30 seconds, the product was washed with ethyl acetate and alcohol to obtain pure compound. Recrystalized from ethanol. Melting point is 202-205°C.

****

Experiment No. 15

Aim: Synthesis of Tetrahydrocarbazole (Borsche–Drechsel cyclization).

Cyclohexane   Phenylhydrazine   1,2,3,4 - tetrahydrocarbazole

A equimolar quantities of cyclohexanone and redistilled phenyl hydrazine was placed in 250 ml round botton flask, with few drops of glacial acetic acid, then subjected to microwave at 320 W for 10 minutes. Then the reaction mixture was cooled to 50°C. The above mixture was filtered at pump and the obtained solid was washed with cold water. Melting point is 115-116°C.

****

Experiment No. 16

Aim: Synthesis of 3H-Quinazolin-4-one (Nimentowski reaction).

Methyl anthranilate   Formamide   3H - quinazoline - 4 - one

5 gm (0.033 mol) of methyl anthranilate and 15 ml of formamide were mixed in 100 ml of two necked round botton flask and subjected to microwave at 350 W for 40 minutes. The reaction mixture was allowed to cool at room temperature and then poured on ice water, the solid separate out was filtered and dried. The crude product on crystallization from methanol-dimethyl formamide mixture yielded 3H-quinazolinone-4-one.

****

(IV) DRAWING STRUCTURES AND REACTIONS USING CHEMDRAW®

ChemDraw also called Chemoffice is one of the softwares used to create chemical structures with ease. This software is much easier for us to have the advantages of drawing a chemical formula. To draw a chemical molecular formula Office includes ChemDraw and 3D. ChemDraw is the chemistry of the product Cabridgesoft.inc software. ChemDraw has many functions, including making the names and structures of compounds and get accurate IUPAC names of the structure. Estimated NMR spectra of a compound structure with direct atom to spectral correlation.

Thus the function of ChemDraw is helpful, ChemDraw is the chemistry of the product Cabridgesoft.inc software. This makes ChemDraw very popular among chemists, especially for chemistry teachers and lecturers because no longer need to describe the chemical structure on the board so as to minimize the time to teach.

A chemical drawing solution that chemists across multiple chemistry disciplines can trust to accurately handle and represent organic, organometallic and polymeric and biopolymer materials (including amino acids, peptides and DNA and RNA sequences) and to deal with advanced forms of stereochemistry.

Chemists who use ChemDraw to predict properties are able to save time and reduce costs by identifying compounds that are likely to have the desired properties before actually synthesizing them.

Chemists can also save time and increase data accuracy using ChemDraw to generate spectra, construct correct IUPAC names, and calculate reaction stoichiometry.

Three different versions of ChemDraw:

- **ChemDraw Ultra**, the newest version of the world's most popular chemical drawing package, contains many exciting new features. Among the highlights of ChemDraw Ultra are the ability to create multipage documents and posters, spectral info to atom correlation in ChemNMR, identification and typing of stereo centers.

ChemDraw Ultra contains.

1.   ChemDraw Ultra Application.

2.   ChemNMR Add-on (NMR Spectral prediction tool).

3.   ChemProp Add-on (Common physical property predictions).

4.   ChemDraw Pro Internet Browser Plugin.

5.   Chem3D Std 8.

6.   Chem3D Std Internet Browser Plugin.

7.   ChemFinder Ultra.

•   **ChemDraw Pro** is the newest release of the most popular chemical drawing program in the world for creating high quality chemical publishing material. It has also become the premier drawing tool for chemical information querying. New features in ChemDraw Pro include ChemProp, SMIRKS support, cross-platform skc file exchange, identify stereo centers.

ChemDraw Pro contains:

1.   ChemDraw Pro Application.

2.   ChemProp Add-on.

3.   ChemDraw Pro Internet Browser Plugin.

4.   Chem3D Std Internet Browser Plugin.

ChemDraw Standard is truly the drawing program for anyone needing to create chemical structure drawings for whatever purpose. It is simple to learn and use and yet offers the novice a wealth of feature options to produce precisely what is needed for the job at hand.

ChemDrawStd contains

1.   ChemDrawStd Application.

2.   ChemDraw Net Internet Browser Plugin.

****

Experiment No. 17

Aim: Drawing Structures and Reactions by using ChemDraw®.

ChemDraw program is developed by David A. Evans and Stewart Rubenstein in 1985, later by the chem informatics company Cambridge Soft. ChemDraw is a simple-to-use program that allows drawing efficiently simple two-dimensional representations of organic molecules. It is available for the PC as well as for the Mac platform. The drawing of chemical formulae and reaction schemes is a repetitive task for chemists on all levels of their education.

ChemDraw is used by all over the world to quickly and effectively draw molecules, reactions and biological pathways for use in documents and electronic lab notebooks.

Features of ChemDraw 12.0:

- Chemical structure to name conversion.
- Chemical name to structure conversion.
- NMR spectrum simulation (^{1}H and ^{13}C).
- Mass spectrum simulation.
- Structure cleanup.

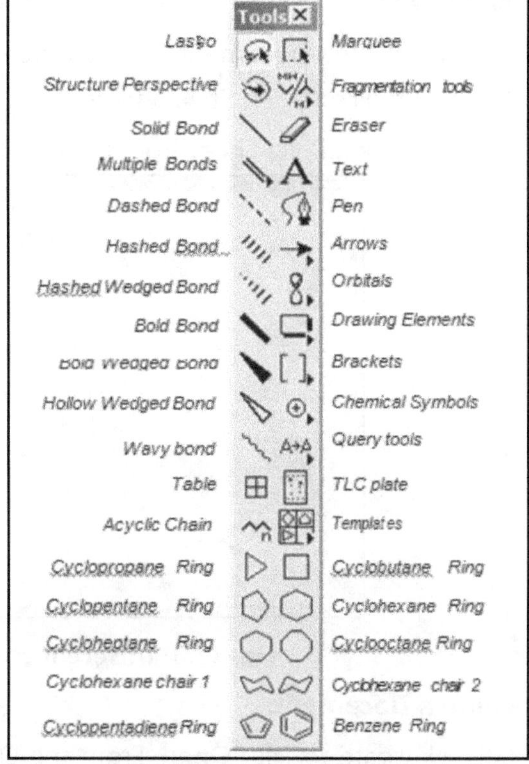

Fig. 17.1: Main Toolbar

ChemDraw Toolbars:

➤ **The Main Toolbar:**

The main toolbar includes the tools used for drawing structures including all selection and bond tools.

➤ **Tearing off Toolbars:**

Tearing off toolbars are indicated by a small black triangle in the lower right corner. For example:

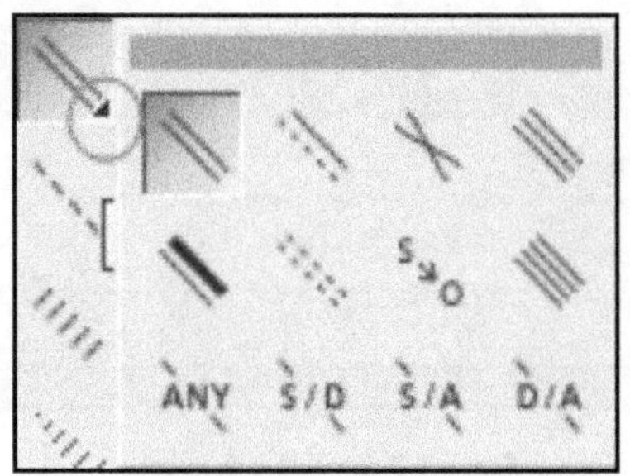

Fig. 17.2: Tearing off Toolbars

Creating a New Document:

To create a document, go to File>New Document.

Using Styles:

➢ To create a new document using a different style sheet or stationery pad:

1. Go to File>Open Style Sheets.

2. Choose a Style Sheet from the list.

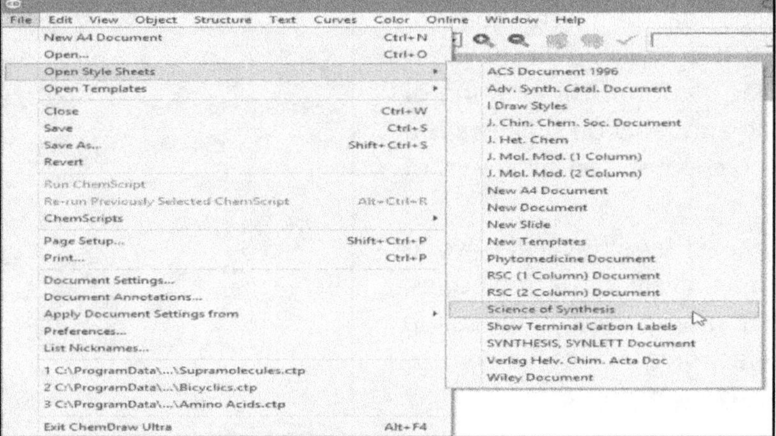

Fig. 17.3: Different style sheet or stationery pad

Opening a Document:

(a) Navigate to File>Open. From the Open dialog, select the file name and location of the file and click Open.

OR

(b) From the File menu, choose the document from the list at the bottom.

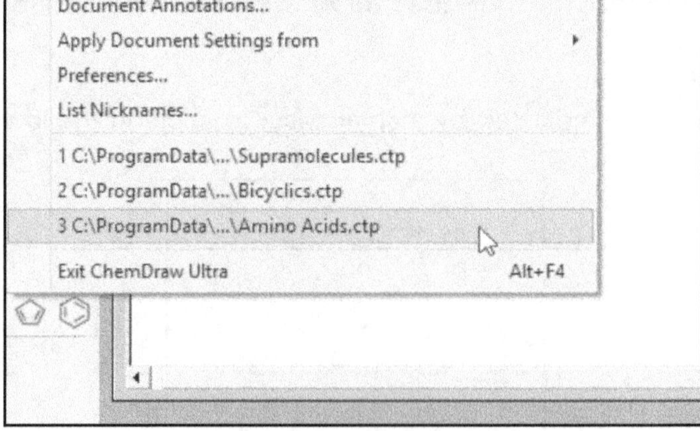

Fig. 17.4: File menu

Table 17.1: Functions of the tools for all versions

Tool	Icon	Explanation
Selection		*Lasso.* Select objects by dragging around them. *Marquee.* Select objects by dragging diagonally across them.
Structure perspective		Rotate a selected object in three dimensions
Fragmentation toolbar		*Fragmentation tool.* Splits molecules across specific bonds. *Dissociation tool.* Breaks bonds and draws a reaction. *Retro synthesis tool.* Breaks bonds and draws a reaction.
Solid bond		Draw bonds and set bond properties.
Eraser		*Delete objects.* Click on an object to delete; drag to delete multiple objects.
Multiple bond toolbar		Draw multiple bonds and set bond properties. Bonds of different types can be selected from the multiple bonds toolbar.
Text		Create atom labels and captions.
Pen		Draw freehand shapes such as custom arrows and orbitals
Arrows toolbar		*Draw arrows.* Arrows of different types can be selected from the arrows toolbar.

Orbitals toolbar		*Draw orbitals.* Orbitals of different types can be selected from the Orbitals toolbar.
Drawing Elements toolbar		Different types of drawing elements can be selected from the Drawing Elements toolbar, such as boxes and lines.
Brackets toolbar		Brackets of different types can be selected from the Brackets toolbar.
Chemical Symbols toolbar		Symbols of different types can be selected from the Symbols tool palette. Draw chemically significant symbols such as charges, radicals and lone pairs.
Acyclic Chain		Draw chains of any length.
Query toolbar		Draw stereochemical flags, indicate free sites, alternative groups and correspondences between atoms in query structures.
Templates toolbars		Draw structures with templates stored in template documents. Templates can be selected from the Templates toolbars.
Rings		Draw common structural components

Chemical Properties Window:

➢ **Chemical Properties view for Methane:**

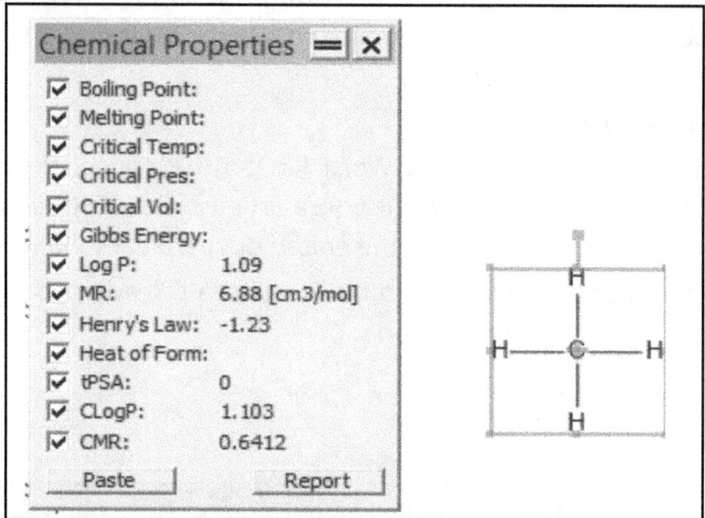

Fig. 17.5: Chemical Properties of Methane

The Analysis Window:

The Analysis window displays the chemical analysis of the selected structure. Window can activate from the View menu.

The Analysis Window View for Methane:

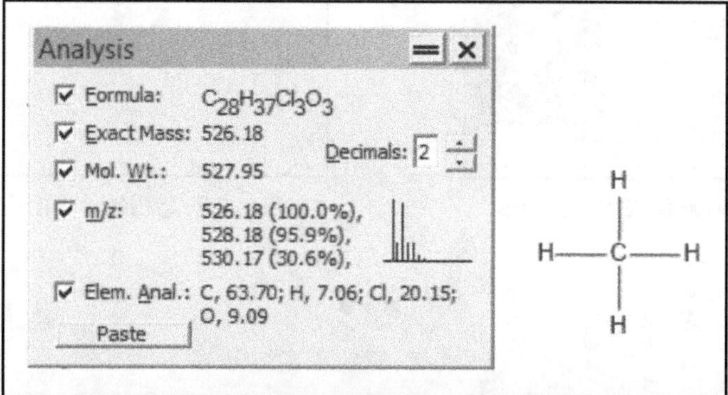

Fig. 17.6: Analysis window for Methane

Importing and Exporting Data from ChemDraw:

- Chemical drawing programs enable scientists to communicate chemical structures.
- ChemDraw includes many of the standard file formats for transferring information between ChemDraw and documents created using other applications.

Exporting Graphics from ChemDraw:

Method 1:

- To insert the ChemDraw. wmf image file into a Microsoft Word document, position the cursor at the appropriate location on the page. Then use INSERT > PICTURE > FROM FILE...
- Select the file and click insert to insert the drawing to the document.

Method 2 (Direct Export Method):

*   To export diagrams from Chem Draw into Word (or other programs): select the diagram, copy it to the clipboard (Edit-Copy or Command-C), go to Word and do Edit-Paste or Command-V to paste it into the document.

Importing Graphics to ChemDraw:

*   Diagrams that have been placed in a Word file can be edited. If double click on the diagram in the Word file, it will extract it into a little window in ChemDraw where it can be edited. Just close the window to put the edited diagram back into the Word file.

*   If right-click on the diagram in the Word file, it will see the edit and open options under the CS ChemDraw Drawing Object option.

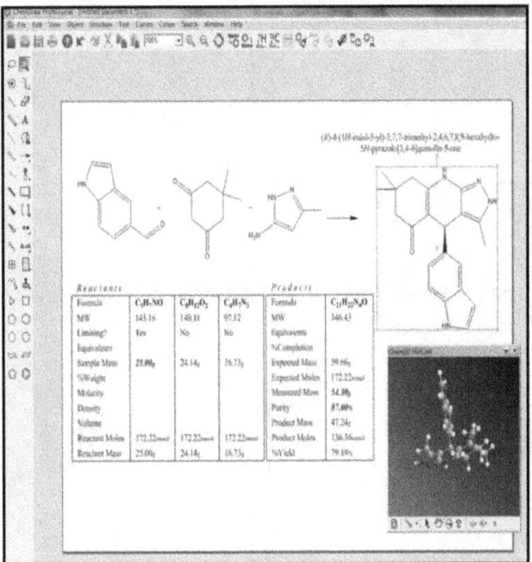

Fig. 17.7: Little window in ChemDraw

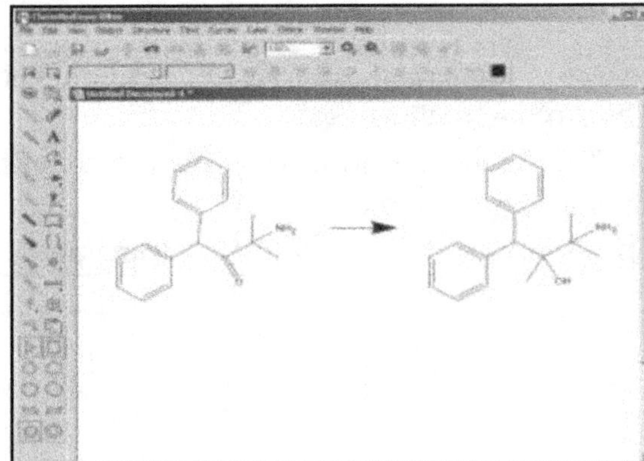

Fig. 17.7: Little window in ChemDraw

✱✱✱

(V) DETERMINATION OF PHYSICOCHEMICAL PROPERTIES SUCH AS LOG P, C LOG P, MR, MOLECULAR WEIGHT, HYDROGEN BOND DONORS AND ACCEPTORS FOR CLASS OF DRUGS COURSE CONTENT USING DRUG DESIGN SOFTWARE DRUG LIKELINESS SCREENING (LIPINSKIES RO5)

Lipinski's rule of five also known as the **Pfizer's rule** of five or simply the **rule of five (RO5)** is a rule of thumb to evaluate drug likeness or determine if a chemical compound with a certain pharmacological or biological activity has chemical properties and physical properties that would make it a likely orally active drug in humans. The rule was formulated by Christopher A. Lipinski in 1997, based on the observation that most orally administered drugs are relatively small and moderately lipophilic molecules.

The rule describes molecular properties important for a drug's pharmacokinetics in the human body, including their absorption, distribution, metabolism, and excretion ("ADME"). However, the rule does not predict if a compound is pharmacologically active.

The rule is important to keep in mind during drug discovery when a pharmacologically active lead structure is optimized step-wise to increase the activity and selectivity of the compound as well as to ensure drug-like physicochemical properties are maintained as described by Lipinski's rule. Candidate drugs that conform to the RO5 tend to have lower attrition rates during clinical trials and hence have an increased chance of reaching the market.

Components of the Rule:

Lipinski's rule states that, in general, an orally active drug has no more than one violation of the following criteria:

- No more than 5 hydrogen bond donors (the total number of nitrogen–hydrogen and oxygen–hydrogen bonds).
- No more than 10 hydrogen bond acceptors (all nitrogen or oxygenatoms).
- A molecular mass less than 500 daltons.
- An octanol-water partition coefficient (log P) that does not exceed 5.

Variants:

- Partition coefficient log P in −0.4 to +5.6 range.
- Molar refractivity from 40 to 130.
- Molecular weight from 180 to 480.
- Number of atoms from 20 to 70 Lead-like.

During drug discovery, lipophilicity and molecular weight are often increased in order to improve the affinity and selectivity of the drug candidate. Hence, it is often difficult to maintain drug-likeness (i.e., RO5 compliance) during hit and lead optimization. Hence, it has been proposed that members of screening libraries from which hits are discovered should be biased toward lower molecular weight and lipophility so that medicinal chemists will have an easier time in delivering optimized drug development candidates that are also drug-like.

***

Experiment No. 18

Aim: To determine molecular properties, Lipinski "Rule of Five" and Bioactivity score.

The data focused on the importance of Lipinski "Rule of Five", Calculation of molecular properties such as log P, polar surface area and number of hydrogen bond donors, number of hydrogen bond acceptors and molecular weight, also prediction of bioactivity score for the most important drug targets like kinase inhibitors, GPCR ligands, ion channel modulators and nuclear receptors.

In the discovery setting 'the rule of 5' predicts that poor absorption is more likely when there are more than 5 H-bond donors, 10 H-bond acceptors and the molecular weight is greater than 500 and the calculated Log P (C Log P) is greater than 5 (or M log P > 4.15). Computational methodology for the rule-based Moriguchi Log P (M Log P) calculation is described. In the development setting, solubility calculations focus on exact value prediction and are difficult because of polymorphism. Useful predictions are possible in closely related analog series when coupled with experimental thermodynamic solubility measurements.

1.1 Lipinski's Rule of Five

Lipinski's rule of five (RO5) is a rule of thumb to evaluate drug likeness or determine if a chemical compound with a certain pharmacological or biological activity has properties that would make it a likely orally active drug in humans. The rule was formulated by Christopher A. Lipinski in 1997, based on the observation that most medication drugs are relatively small and lipophilic molecules. The rule describes molecular properties important for a drug's pharmacokinetics in the human body, including their absorption, distribution, metabolism, and excretion. However, the rule does not predict if a compound is pharmacologically active.

The rule is important to keep in mind during drug discovery when a pharmacologically active lead structure is optimized step-wise to increase the activity and selectivity of the compound as well as to insure drug-like physicochemical properties are maintained as described by Lipinski's rule.

1.1.1 Components of the Rule

- Not more than 5 hydrogen bond donors (nitrogen or oxygen atoms with one or more hydrogen atoms).
- Not more than 10 hydrogen bond acceptors (nitrogen or oxygen atoms).
- A molecular mass less than 500 daltons.
- An octanol-water partition coefficient log P not greater than 5.

1.1.2 Variants

- Partition coefficient log P in −0.4 to +5.6 range.
- Molar refractivity from 40 to 130.

- Molecular weight from 180 to 500.

- Number of atoms from 20 to 70 (includes H-bond donors [e.g. OH's and NH's] and H-bond acceptors [e.g.; N's and O's]).

- Polar surface area no greater than 140 Å^2.

Also the 500 molecular weight cutoff has been questioned. Polar surface area and the number of rotatable bonds has been found to better discriminate between compounds that are orally active and those that are not for a large data set of compounds. In particular, compounds which meet only the two criteria of:

- 10 or fewer rotatable bonds.

- Polar surface area equal to or less than 140 Å^2 are predicted to have good oral bioavailability.

1.1.3 Lead-like

During drug discovery, lipophilicity and molecular weight are often increased in order to improve the affinity and selectivity of the drug. Hence, it is often difficult to maintain drug-likeness (i.e. RO5 compliance) during hit and lead optimization. Hence, it has been proposed that members of screening libraries from which hits are discovered should be biased towards lower molecular weight and lipophility so that medicinal chemists will have an easier time in delivering optimized drug development candidates that are also drug-like.

Hence, the rule of five has been extended to the rule of three (RO3) for defining lead-like compounds.

A rule of three compliant compounds is defined as one that has:

- Octanol-water partition coefficient log P not greater than 3.

- Molecular mass less than 300 daltons.

- Not more than 3 hydrogen bond donors.

- Not more than 3 hydrogen bond acceptors.

- Not more than 3 rotatable bonds.

This is best explained using the below graphical representation in Fig. 18.1 of chemical space. It is introduced by Lipinski and Hopkins where compounds are mapped onto coordinates of chemical descriptors of physicochemical properties. For example, it is known that active site inhibitors for protease families cluster together in a discrete region of chemical space.

The intersection of this cluster with the descriptor space for drug-like compounds would contain in this example the protease inhibitors that have the potential to be developed as oral drugs. Such an overlap would allow the conclusion that the protease family is druggable. The most challenging part of a protease inhibitor optimization is changing a peptidic lead compound into an orally bioavailable peptidomimetic. This step has proven to be relatively straightforward for some proteases (e.g. thrombin), whereas for others it may be an almost impossible job due to the amino acid content of the lead and the shallowness of the binding pocket.

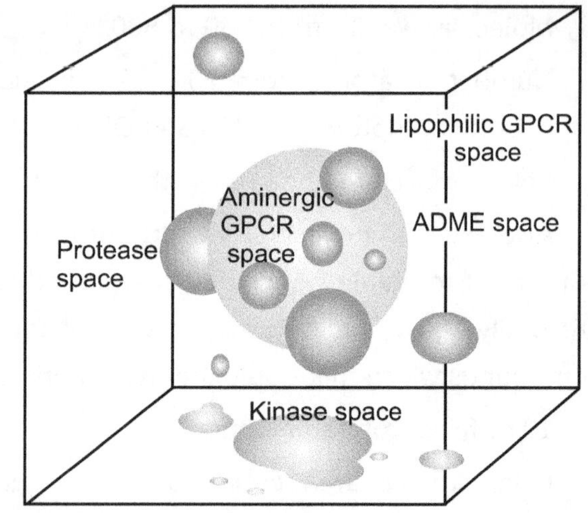

Fig. 18.1: Representation of the relationship between the continuums of chemical space

A graphical representation of the relationship between the continuum of chemical space (light blue) and the discrete areas occupied by compounds with specific affinity for certain protein classes. The independent intersection of compounds with drug-like properties is shown in green. The second step of quantitatively assessing the druggability of the identified pockets is more challenging. An obvious approach is to screen a large library of drug-like compounds. Unfortunately, this approach has three significant drawbacks i.e. it is very expensive, applied rather late in the drug discovery process and it produces a large number of false positives hits which complicate the analysis.

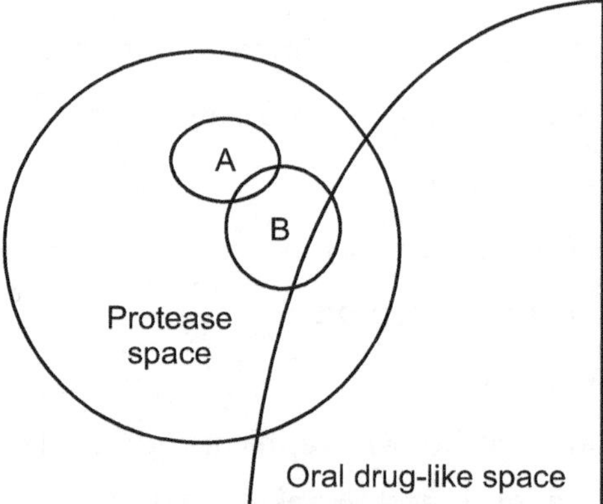

Fig. 18.2: Chemical space occupied by active site serine protease inhibitors

Fig. 18.2 shows that the chemical space occupied by active site serine protease inhibitors. Since, this bubble intersects with the oral drug-like space, we would come to the conclusion that the serine protease family is druggable. The situation is, however, more complex. Some serine proteases will be druggable whereas others are not.

1.1.4 Conclusion on RO5

The RO5 and it's extensions have been useful tools to generate awareness about the importance of PK parameters for development. In addition, this concept has led to the realization that there may be whole families of proteins for which it is either extremely challenging to design compounds with good oral bioavailability.

The available evidence suggests that qualitative druggability arguments are useful strategic tools; however, more accurate, quantitative assessments are needed. This is a very attractive approach that can be used in the early stages of drug discovery and provides a solid basis for computational druggability estimations. It has been suggested that the inability of the pharmaceutical industry to solve druggability problems is due to limitations in current medicinal chemistry approaches. Druggability is defined by molecular properties and therefore it is unlikely that advances in synthesis, profiling or innovative design will solve these problems.

The real druggability challenge arrives when these 'leads' have to be turned into orally bioavailable, pharmaceutically useful drug candidates. It has never been challenging to make inhibitors of proteins with questionable druggability, but rather the challenge has been to make orally bioavailable, pharmaceutically useful inhibitors that successfully advance through clinical development. It is likely that oral drugs for the modulation of such proteins will continue to come from the natural-product pool. In addition, future advances in drug delivery may offer solutions to address problems of druggability.

✱✱✱

OUT UPCOMING BOOKS
As Per PCI Regulations Third Year (Semester VI)

- **Medicinal Chemistry III :** S.G. Walode
- **Medicinal Chemistry III :** K.G. Bothara
- **Practical Medicinal chemistry III :** S.G. Walode
- **Pharmacology III :** Dr. S. V. Tembhurne
- **Pharmacology III :** K.G. Bothara
- **Practical Pharmacology III :** Dr. Arjun Patra
- **Herbal Drug Technology :** Vaibhav shinde, Ms. K. S. Bodas, S.B. Gokhale
- **Practical Herbal Drug Technology :** Vaibhav Shinde, Ms. K. S. Bodas, S.B. Gokhale
- **Biopharmaceutics and Pharmacokinetics :** Sunil bakliwal
- **Pharmaceutical Biotechnology :** Dr. Chandrakant Kokare
- **Medicinal Chemistry III :** Dr. Abhishek Tiwari
- **Pharmacology III :** Dr. Rupesh Gautam, Dr. Kalpesh Gour
- **Herbal Drug Technology :** Dr. Versha Tiwari, Dr. Vikash Sharma
- **Biopharmaceutics and Pharmacokinetics :** Hari Kumar
- **Pharmaceutical Biotechnology :** Dr. Khush Yadav, Mr. Rajiv Saxena, Ms. Satinder Kaur, Garima Joshi
- **Quality Assurance :** Bhupender Sing Tomar, Dr. Pawan Jhalwal, Surajpal verma
- **Medicinal Chemistry III :** Vibha Chandan Patil, Dr Chandrashekhar Narajji
- **Medicinal Chemistry III :** Mr. Mayur S. Jain, Mr. Mayur R. Bhurat, Sanjay A. Nagdev, Dr. Md. Rageeb Md. Usman
- **Practical Medicinal Chemistry III :** Dr. Sunita T. Patil, Dr. Md. Rageeb Md. Usman, Dr. Parloop A. Bhatt
- **Pharmacology III :** Dr. Manjunatha. P. Mudagal
- **Practical Pharmacology III :** Dr. Manjunatha. P. Mudagal
- **Herbal Drug Technology :** Kuntal Das
- **Herbal Drug Technology :** Dr. Santram Lodhi, Dr. Md. Rageeb Md. Usman, Dr. Tushar A. Deshmukh, Mr. Vaibhav M. Darvhekar
- **Practical Herbal Drug Technology :** Prof. Md. Rageeb Md. Usman, Prof. Vaibhav M. Darvhekar, Prof. (Dr.) Akhila S., Prof. (Dr.) Vijay Kumar D.
- **Biopharmaceutics and Pharmacokinetics :** Dr. B. Prakash Rao
- **Pharmaceutical Biotechnology :** Kuntal Das
- **A Practical Book Of Medicinal Chemistry (Combined Book Sem. IV & VI)** Dr. Abhishek Tiwari, Dr. Rajeev Kumar

****

www.ingramcontent.com/pod-product-compliance
Lightning Source LLC
Chambersburg PA
CBHW082006160726
47999CB00008B/2730